NEW BOOK ON SEX EDUCATION

Understanding Sex, Sexuality and Improving Sexual Relationships

Table of Contents

Chapter 1

Introduction to sex

Sex is one of the most overused and overused terms in today's language. Therefore, it is vital to ask "what is sex" because it might imply different things to different people.

When discussing the act of having sex, it simply refers to someone taking pleasure in and participating in an intimate encounter with their partner, which may involve foreplay, snuggling, kissing, hugging, and penetration. Sex is varied for many sexual orientations.
While starting the path toward a deeper understanding of sex, one of the first lessons you need to learn is to let go of all the taboos associated with the idea of having sex and

accept it as an expression of love and passion.

People engage in sexual activity for a variety of reasons. For some, it is motivated by an innate desire or lust, while for others, it is a means of reproduction. Similarly to this, some individuals could only value physical closeness with someone they truly love. What sex means to you will therefore likely be strongly influenced by what arouses you and by what you enjoy or dislike when engaged in any sexual activity. Recall that while "intercourse" is the definition of sex, it does not only refer to "penetrative sex" or "coitus," but rather to everything that seems sexual.

The simple and obvious question of what is sex becomes relevant and crucial when we consider the crippling status of sex education in our nation. Sex is a love-based, consensual act; if one party is unwilling to participate, it is rape rather than sex.

Understanding the dynamics of sex, what it includes, the problems it raises, and one's sexual preferences is complicated.
Oftentimes, especially when one is young and inexperienced, it can be challenging to comprehend one's feelings regarding sex.

Is this subject that gives you the creeps? You're unaware of your potential sex preferences? Are you prepared to have sex? When should a person have their first sexual experience? Sex is painful? We examine the topic and make an effort to respond to all of these questions to address those that are relevant to it.

WHAT IS SEX?
As was already mentioned, different people's definitions of sex might vary. It can be influenced by how you were raised, your views, your sexual orientation, and even your gender because it is now being studied how differently men and women view sex.

Other than vaginal sex, a sexual act may not even entail vaginal sex at all. It includes anything and everything that feels sexual, including kissing, hugging, and any kind of sexually charged touch. It also includes anal sex, oral sex, stripping in front of someone, and so on. Yet, the definition of sex states that it is an act of penetration or intercourse.

TYPES OF SEX
As was previously stated, the act of intercourse and penetration is all that sex is inherently about. Yet, when we discuss the various forms of sex, we typically refer to the various forms of sexual activity, which can include the following sorts.

Vaginal sex
This type of heteronormative, straight sex involves a man inserting his penis into a woman's vagina. The most typical kind of sex is this.

Even though studies indicate that all women are either bisexual or gay but not straight, there is still relatively little recognition of this fact.

Oral sex
By swallowing them or licking them, you might verbally arouse your partner's sexual organs. Oral sexual activity can be engaged in by partners with any sexual interest and is not sexual orientation specific.

Anal Sex
It alludes to getting into a partner's anus. Anal sex is typically associated with gay males, but more and more women are increasingly engaging in it. Anal intercourse entails a number of extra dangers in addition to an increased risk of infection.

Mutual Masturbation
There is no penetration involved in this type of intercourse.

It entails masturbating in front of or assisting your spouse in masturbating. The risk of STDs, pregnancy, or illnesses is completely eliminated with this type of sexual activity, making it the safest.

Health Benefits of Sex
There are many health advantages of sex. Here is a list of them:

❖ Sexual activity boosts immunological function.

You will require fewer and fewer sick days if you are sexually healthy and active. This is due to the fact that having sex helps you build up your immunity, which will reduce the number of times you get the flu or a cold. This is because having sex causes your body's antibody levels to rise. You must engage in sexual activity once or twice per week in order to boost your immunity.

❖ lowers elevated blood pressure

possess hypertension? Have a sexual encounter. You may think that this is the most avant-garde piece of advice you have heard so far, but there is a good explanation for it. Regular sexual activity and decreased blood pressure have been linked in studies. According to a study, sex alone—not even masturbation—helped reduce systolic blood pressure.

❖ Sexual activity increases libido

In essence, this is claiming that a man becomes flawless via practice.
Your libido increases as you have more sex, making it even more fantastic. In particular, for women, having more sex improves their sex because it increases their vaginal lubrication, suppleness, and blood flow in those areas.

❖ Sex aids in improving bladder control in women.

30% of women have incontinence at some point in their life. They can manage their incontinence if they engage in regular sex since it strengthens their pelvic muscles.

They are primarily made stronger by orgasms since they cause contractions in those muscles, which in turn strengthen them.

❖ Sex expends energy.

You didn't work out today. Forget it. Have a sexual encounter. This is due to the tremendous benefits of sex as exercise. Certain challenging and physically demanding positions can burn up to 300 calories! The general consensus is that one minute of sex will burn five calories. This indicates that a session lasting 30 minutes can burn roughly 150 calories.

❖ Sexual activity enhances heart health

The hormones estrogen and testosterone will remain under control if you engage in regular sexual activity. The risk of osteoporosis and heart disease is reduced when they are kept in your body in the proper proportion. According to a study, guys who have sex twice a week had a 50% lower risk of dying from a heart attack than men who only have sex occasionally.

❖ Prostate cancer risk is decreased by sex.

According to a study, males who ejaculate more frequently than five times per week, or over 20 times per month, have a lower risk of developing prostate cancer. Whilst the ejaculation may be caused by masturbation or even nocturnal discharge, this isn't always about having sex.

❖ Pain can be numb by sex.

assuming you had an orgasm. Because it produces a hormone that might lower your pain threshold, orgasm is referred to as a natural pain blocker or killer.
In fact, it can also block the discomfort and lessen menstrual cramps, headaches, leg pain, and even arthritic pain—but only if you vaginally stimulate yourself.

❖ Sex eases tension

Your body produces feel-good hormones during sex, which relieves stress and anxiety. It may even improve your relationship's intimacy and help you feel better about yourself.

❖ Sex improves sleep quality.

The hormone prolactin is released in your body during an orgasm.

As soon as you have sex, it can greatly calm you and aid in your ability to fall asleep.

❖ It may increase your partner's level of intimacy.

Sex is a powerful tool for building a strong bond with your partner. According to studies, having sex increases a couple's intimacy, dependence on one another, and trust level.

What you need right now might be sex!

The long-term solution is not sex, we frequently say. It might not be one, but what if all you require right now is a temporary solution?

THE CRITICAL ROLE OF FOREPLAY IN SEX

Not engaging in foreplay at all or not for long enough before sex is a mistake that many individuals make. There is a common misconception that only women require foreplay. That is not the case, though. Engaging in foreplay can greatly improve even men's sexual lives.

Foreplay has a ton of advantages. Foreplay is a terrific way to build physical and emotional intimacy as well as better sex. According to studies, engaging in appropriate foreplay with your spouse lengthens your sessions and improves the climax. Allowing yourself sufficient arousal is crucial, even if you're masturbating, as it might affect the quality of your orgasm and your level of satisfaction.

DO'S AND DON'T DO'S DURING SEX

Both men and women have certain bedtime preferences.
You'll probably have the best sexual life if you go about them in the right manner. Are you curious about your guy's preferences? Here are some suggestions for appropriate

and inappropriate behavior when dating a
man.

- ❖ Be assertive and direct. Guys adore
  partners who are willing to go all in
  and are self-assured enough to make
  direct requests.

- ❖ Give him the finger. Guys enjoy seeing
  things, thus visual stimulation is the
  best they can hope for.

- ❖ Be assured. Everyone has concerns
  about the way their bodies seem, as we
  all know. It's normal to not feel very
  confident with your hairy thighs or the
  scar on your back. Everything will be
  OK if you have confidence.

- ❖ Rule over your man. He appreciates it
  when you grab the reins.

And most importantly, express your fantasies to others. He will be more forthcoming about them the more honest you are with him. Sex is always nice when you and your partner talk about your likes and dislikes, what you would like, and other topics.

- ❖ Don't discuss babies. Indeed, it may be what is going through your thoughts, but try to enjoy the act of sex in the present rather than thinking about starting a family when you could be orgasming.

- ❖ Avoid calling his penis "cute," as that can put him under pressure and be a major letdown.

❖ Never appear drowsy or bored. He wants to see that you are intrigued by him.

❖ Avoid speaking too much. While you don't have to refrain from sexual grousing, you should avoid bringing up topics like your best friend's crush or the reasons you despise your coworker.

❖ Never, ever pretend to have an orgasm.

We now examine what women desire and do not desire in sex.

❖ You must speak loudly, curse, and grunt. They adore it.

❖ She should be touched all over with your hands. Don't simply pay attention to the two major organs; consider the entire body.

❖ Undress her. When you do it, she enjoys it.

❖ Observe her closely. Are you a fan of "Game of Thrones"? If so, you are aware of how crucial it is to maintain eye contact throughout sexual activity.

❖ Do not attempt to give her harsh friction by treating her clitoris. Try to be as kind as you can.

❖ emit sound. Speak and act verbally. Tell her what you want and whether something appeals to you.

❖ Never skip the foreplay. You shouldn't assume that a little 10-second kiss will be enough to make a woman swoon.

THE VALUE OF ORGASM
When we have sex, our goal is to experience orgasms. Orgasming has a ton of advantages, many of which have already been highlighted.

You should nevertheless be aware of the various orgasms and how to use them.
Orgasms can be explosive or implosive, or they can release or absorb energy, respectively. Men are typically thought to experience explosive orgasms, whereas women are thought to have implosive orgasms.

There is no denying the significance of orgasms. Orgasm is an extremely potent energy that can improve relationships, boost immunity, and reduce stress.

Chapter 2

Sex position

Sex positions can be rather perplexing unless you've done extensive reading on the Kama Sutra or something comparable. How then can you decide which position you want to try out next when they all seem so intimidating and challenging? Don't worry, the most popular sex positions are listed below along with their advantages and disadvantages.

❖ Missionary

It functions as the most typical sex position. Your spouse is on top of you as you lay on your back with your legs spread wide.

Benefits: It's the ideal job for newcomers. You can look at each other and kiss. You can also treat one another with kindness.

Cons: Eventually, it just becomes boring. Lack of effort results in dissatisfaction.

❖ Doggy Style

Doggy style is when you are on all fours and your partner is grabbing hold of you from behind while he is kneeling.

Positives: Your companion will love the vista! Also, it's simple to access your clitoris from behind.

Cons: If your partner enters too forcefully, it might be a little unpleasant; some people even think it's a beastly position.

❖ Cowgirl

The standard "female on top" sex position is how it functions. You sit or kneel over your companion as he lies on his back and, well, ride him!

Pros: If you want to induce vaginal orgasms, this is a terrific sex position for you. Also, it enables your boyfriend to further titillate you with his hands. Your first action toward sex dominance is unquestionably correct!

Cons: If done improperly, leaves the partner with little to do and frequently results in being a turnoff.

❖ The 69

How it functions This position resembles the number "69" quite a bit. Both lovers are in a top-to-tail position, either on top of or by their sides. The mouths are what make contact with and manipulate their partner's genitalia.

Pros: While not being intercourse in the strictest sense of the word, position 69 is fantastic for arousal!

Cons: It takes time and practice to become proficient in this position. You should put more effort into giving yourself and your lover pleasure.

❖ Face to Face

You face each other, link your legs behind him, and crawl onto his lap.

Advantages: It's a wonderfully cuddly posture that almost feels like sex. Also, you have the opportunity to work toward the climax together.

Cons: The process is incredibly slow, which may not be to everyone's taste.

❖ Spoons

How it operates: Essentially, spooning with sex. Your lover approaches you from behind while you both lie with your backs to the same side, forming the shape of two spoons coming together.

Positives: This is a fairly tranquil and laid-back position. Great for couples who genuinely like being around one another.

Cons: It's not for those who enjoy intense sex and are attracted to its provocative nature.

❖ The Scissors

Scissors is a simple pose to perform, though it may be a little difficult to describe. He pulls you by your butt and enters you when you both turn to face each other and place your top leg over your partner.

Pros: This position's intimacy is incredibly captivating! When you are just a few inches apart, you can kiss your companion. not even inches, perhaps.

Cons: It's not very aesthetically appealing and it takes a few tries to get it perfect.

❖ Galloping Horse

You'll need a chair for this one to operate. One is where your lover sits, and the other is where you climb up to ignite your passion.

Pros: Your lover is attracted to your attractive view. You also receive deep penetration!

Cons: Doing it while sitting in a chair can occasionally be challenging, and maintaining your legs apart can be very uncomfortable.

❖ Magic Bullet

How it works: Your partner kneels behind you and holds onto your knees for leverage and thrusts as you lie face up on the bed with your legs straight up in the air.

Pros: Just like the last position, this one's movements are sensual and deep, truly living up to the title!

Cons: It might be very exhausting if you're not into working out. You can have sore legs the next day.

❖ Corridor Canoodling

How it works is simple: You and your partner must locate a space with two walls that are directly opposite one another. While you climb on top of him, your partner leans against one wall, putting his feet against the other.

Advantages: It's ideal for quickies or toilet sex. It's fun and impulsive at the same time!

Cons: To carry your weight while also attempting to make the most of the situation, your partner would need to have strong legs.

❖ Reverse Cowgirl

How it functions: It combines dog style and woman-on-top, and it is the antithesis of cowgirl. With their legs hanging over the side of the bed, your companion is lying flat. You climb on top of your partner, but turn your back on him. You then bend forward and lay your arms on his knees or thighs.

Pros: You have complete control over the movement's speed, angle, and direction!

Cons: Couples often prefer more physical interaction, but there is very little of it here.

Chapter 3

What phases make up the sexual response cycle?

The sexual response cycle contains four distinct phases:

Desire (libido).
Arousal(excitement).
Orgasm.
Resolution.

Though the timing may differ, both men and women may be affected by these periods. For instance, it's rare for two partners to have an orgasm at the same time. The intensity of the response and the length of each phase also vary from person to person. Women don't always go through the sexual phases in this particular order.

Some of these stages may not occur or may occur out of order during some sexual situations. Some people may be motivated by a need for intimacy to engage in sexual behavior. If partners are better able to understand one another's bodies and reactions, the sexual experience may be enhanced.

Over the many stages of sexual engagement, there may be numerous physiologic changes. Individuals may experience some, all, or none of these changes.

1st Stage: Desire
These are some common characteristics of this phase, which may last over a short period of time or for a very long time:

The muscles become tenser.
Heart rate rises and breathing becomes more rapid.
The skin may become flushed (blotches of redness may appear on the chest and back).

Nipples harden or become erect.

Increased blood flow to the genitals is what causes the swelling of a woman's clitoris and labia minora (inner lips) and the erection of a man's penis.

Vaginal lubrication can begin.

The woman's breasts enlarge, and the vaginal walls begin to bulge.

The man's testicles become larger, his scrotum tightens, and he begins to secrete lubricant.

It's important to keep in mind that every person has a different sexual experience. The aforementioned modifications might not have always been apparent to everyone. This may vary not only between various individuals but even within an individual over the course of multiple sexual encounters. There are times when the period of desire comes after arousal.

2nd Stage: Arousal

The general characteristics of this phase, which lasts till the approach of orgasm, are as follows:

The initial changes of the first phase become more pronounced.
When the blood flow increases and the vagina continues to grow, the vaginal walls get darker.
The woman grows a clitoris that is incredibly sensitive (may even be painful to touch).
The subject, a guy, raises his testicles into his scrotum.

Blood pressure, pulse rate, and breathing all keep rising.
Muscular spasms might start in the hands, face, or feet.
The muscles become tenser.

3rd stage: Orgasm
The sexual response cycle peaks at this stage. It usually just lasts a few seconds and is the quickest of the phases. The following are some general characteristics of this phase:

Muscle contractions that are not voluntary start.
The heartbeat, respiration, blood pressure, and oxygen intake are all at their greatest rates.
Feet muscles tense up.
Sexual tension is released abruptly and strongly.
The muscles in the vagina contract in females. Moreover, the uterus may experience regular contractions.
The ejaculation of semen occurs when the muscles at the base of the penis in men contract rhythmically.
A "sex flush" or rash may develop all over the body.

Final Stage: Resolution
The body gradually resumes its regular level of functioning during this phase, and swollen and erect bodily parts shrink back to their original size and color. Some people have a general sense of well-being and frequent exhaustion throughout this time. With more sexual stimulation, some women can return quickly to the orgasm phase and perhaps have numerous orgasms. After orgasm, men often require a "refractory interval," in which they are unable to experience orgasm once more. Each person's refractory period lasts a different amount of time, and it changes as they become older.

Chapter 4

Using sex toys in your relationship: How to do it

Exploring sex toys with partners doesn't have to be a scary or challenging task.

All parties involved may experience completely new levels of pleasure when sex toys are used during partner sex.

Toys can vibrate and pulse in ways that our bodies can't. Many people can benefit from these unique feelings by having orgasmic experiences that are more regular, frequent, complicated, or intense. Also, the sheer diversity of experiences available to couples can keep their sexual encounters fresh and fascinating, which undoubtedly contributes to the maintenance of desire in long-term partnerships.

Looks good, doesn't it? Although there are fewer taboos surrounding the use of sex toys in general, many people are still hesitant to bring toys into the bedroom with partners.

Why do we hesitate to use sex toys with partners, then?
The reluctance is frequently caused, at least in part, by ingrained notions that sex is about two individuals satisfying each other's physical needs while toys are for solo play.

Marketing that presents toys as substitutes for absent partners or fixes for sexual issues is ineffective. It causes people to perceive interest in toys as an assault on their sexual performance or as sexual competition, especially straight cis guys who rarely play with toys. (They most certainly are not.) People constantly fear coming across as strange, so rather than upset the status quo, they "assume, 'this is what this person enjoys in sex,' and continue the course forever," according to one author.

How to have better sex as well as the sex toy conversations we want to have
Exploring sex toys with partners doesn't have to be a scary or challenging task. Recently, a dozen sex counselors, educators, and toy specialists revealed some essential pointers and strategies for bringing up the subject effectively and pleasantly.

Think about the time
These professionals stated that trying to simply pull out toys during sex is one of the major blunders people make when trying to introduce them to their partners. This can leave your partner feeling anxious and pushed, possibly bringing up fears or causing disagreement, unless you are confident that they are at ease with you and enjoy surprises during sex.

Instead, schedule some time away from sex to discuss and include toys in your play. In a brand-new relationship, it's simple to do. Ideally, at that time, you'll already be discussing your sexual preferences in public and can easily incorporate toys into those conversations. Yet, discussing sexual preferences requires a level of openness that not everyone finds comfortable at first. Even those who do might not feel or think they can bring up toys directly in early conversations.

And it's all right. In a relationship, there is never a good time to bring up sex toys. You can bring up toys months or even years from now, once you've begun having more frequent and open discussions about your sexual needs and desires. Toys could be a fantastic starting point to start a more intimate chat if you've never had one before. If you're unsure of how to approach that first conversation, try framing it as an idea you came across in a piece of writing, online discussion, or in chat with a buddy.

Never be critical or sorry.
Try not to explicitly link your interest in toys to a critique or displeasure with the sex you're presently having, no matter when or how you initiate the subject. That will directly feed into whatever underlying anxieties your partner could have.

Also, avoid making excuses or holding back on your desires because doing so will only serve to increase tension and stress on either one or both sides of the debate. Instead, consider approaching your relationship from a point of discovery, where sex toys are just one of the fun things you can do together to explore what you can add to your sex life and create wonderful new experiences. Most of us are eager to seek out more intense forms of pleasure with our partners because we want them to enjoy themselves during sex.

Don't push the concept.
Do not impose demands or ultimatums on your partner if they are not receptive to the discussion or the concept. Instead, attempt to discuss why that thought makes them uncomfortable, and then look for later methods to address any stigmas or worries they might have about toys or sex.

Be receptive to the notion of exploration.
Try not to dictate what that will look like, including the toys you're going to use together and how you're going to use them if your partner is interested in exploring the potential of toys. Instead, continue discussing the types of sensations you both like or are interested in exploring in that first conversation and later on, as well as how you might see toys enhancing the sex you already have. Urge one another to

consider genital stimulation in novel ways. Discuss how your ideas overlap or diverge. You can start to immerse yourself more thoroughly in toys once you have that understanding.

You or your spouse may already own one or more toys that you or they use on your own but are eager to try out together. When this happens, the partner who has the toy should bring it into bed at a certain time, show their partner how to use it on themselves, and then either physically or vocally prompt them to join in, or instruct them on how to attempt to use the toy on or with each other.

Also, you might want to look at brand-new toys as a pair to find something that complements your special dynamic. You might make looking up and purchasing toys a date activity for you two, giving you the chance to deepen your connection and experience shared anticipation. Leigh, though, advises against falling prey to the temptation of only looking into gadgets designed for couples. Online resources abound, some of which are supported by professionals in sexual health. But, they cannot be relied upon in any manner to be more effective for couples than any other toys.

In reality, many are designed with assumptions about the anatomy of their users to simultaneously stimulate both. The same form of stimulation seldom serves two people simultaneously, and many people find that using a toy on their partner, watching them use a toy, or engaging in mutual masturbation with two distinct toys is more enjoyable than the available two-party stimulations.

Be careful.
Every toy has the potential to be a couple's toy. Of all, there are so many toys available

that the choice might be overwhelming. Keep in mind that there is no rush. Take your time and jointly consider your options: Before purchasing one or more toys, research methods to use them by reading toy reviews, speaking with friends and professionals, and buying them.

On how couples can utilize different toys, some publications have issued what appear to be definitive recommendations. But as long as you're acting safely (i.e., avoiding insertive play with toys that don't have flared bases and using plenty of toy-safe lubrication), you get to choose the rules. That is appropriate for you if it feels wonderful to you.

Also, enjoy it
Being able to laugh at the toy and yourself will help you cope with the inevitable failure of some of your trials. Toys are not inexpensive, so this might be irritating. Yet,

you can find helpful instructions online for practical, body-safe devices that will enable you to play lengthy rounds of exploration with a partner without spending a fortune.

And keep in mind that even when things don't go as planned or perfectly, it's all a part of the trip you're on with your spouse and can help you get closer.

Chapter 5

Importance of Sex and Sexual health

We live in a sex-negative culture with no actual sex education, which makes taking care of your sexual health difficult, strange, and fascinating.
The concept of sexual health has several diverse components. I want to discuss pleasure, a crucial aspect of sex and sexual health that even in-depth sex education typically ignores. Here are some key concepts you need to know.

Exploring sexuality is a continuous process. There are many moving elements to sexuality, including the people you are attracted to, the things that turn you on, the things you are inquisitive about, your boundaries, and more. Your sexuality will evolve throughout time, just like how your taste in food changes with time—it's a never-ending process. Permit yourself to investigate this novel perspective on your body and self.

Understanding your body as a source of pleasure entails doing this. Decide what makes you feel good: Where does touching oneself feel pleasant when/if you do it? What pressure and movements? What goes through your mind when you're awake?

Context, as well as where and how you're being touched, can play just as big of a role in what makes you turn on. Some people find it difficult to enjoy sex when they're anxious or untrusting about their partner. Exploring your sexuality involves learning what you need to truly feel pleasure.

Of course, a lot of people have complex attitudes toward both their bodies and sex. You may experience shame related to sex and sexuality, gender dysphoria, disability, or body image issues. You might have endured sexual assault or abuse. You should not feel compelled to engage in sexual activity (either alone or with a partner) or sexual exploration before you are fully prepared. Consider speaking with a therapist if you're finding it difficult to cope with your feelings or the things you've been through. They can assist you in overcoming it.

Every person experiences pleasure differently.
Porn, films, and television programs typically only present a small selection of physical kinds, sex acts, relationships, and sexualities. But the reverse is true. You are as unique as your sexuality. There is NO justification for feeling ashamed of your level of arousal (or turned on). Hips being caressed, nipples being rubbed, ears being licked, or feet being massaged may be enjoyable to some people while being abhorrent to others. Each body is unique,

and that is not only acceptable but also kind
of amazing!

PIV intercourse is frequently portrayed as
the (ahem) crème de la crème of sexual
activity. As a result, many clitorises
experience confusion or embarrassment
when they are unable to exit PIV. Also,
LGBTQ people are completely excluded
from the discussion. However, most clitoris
sufferers can't or hardly ever experience
orgasms through PIV intercourse on their
own. They frequently require clitoral
stimulation directly. It can come from
fingers, a tongue, a vibrating toy, or
something else.

As diverse as people's bodies are, so too are
their imaginations and passions. It's
probably not unusual if you have a fantasy
or hobby that you consider to be so. People
are interested in various kinds of topics,
after all. The most important thing is that

having sex leaves you and your partner feel safe and healthy and is entirely consensual.

The following scenarios, however, should be avoided: paying for sex, having intercourse with a very young person, having sex in public or with a teacher, and many others.

Don't be frightened to speak up.
In terms of sexual health, communication is crucial—and not just because it's necessary to discuss condoms, STIs, and birth control. Also, it's crucial to discuss your interests and those of your partner. You may establish boundaries and discover your partner's boundaries by being open with them. Decide what you DO NOT want to do, then communicate this to your spouse. Find out your partner's "hard no"s by asking them.

It is not acceptable to disregard a partner's boundaries, put pressure on them, or make them feel bad about the boundaries they have established. This might even constitute sexual assault in some situations. Never take a partner's cooperation for granted just because they haven't objected. Consent must be given voluntarily and explicitly.

It's okay if sex isn't your thing.
If you're not interested in having sex, that's perfectly acceptable and natural. As you age, you can develop an interest in something, or you might not. Whatever you decide, do you.

Asking inquiries is a wonderful thing.
Being at ease with your body and sexuality can help you enjoy yourself more, which is crucial for many people. To be intrigued about sex (or not to be curious!) is completely normal. Ask questions if you're curious about sex, sexuality, or your body! Speak to someone you can trust. It's fantastic if you feel at ease speaking with one of your parents. If not, you can speak with a medical professional, a member of your family (such as an aunt, cousin, or

brother), or a friend. But, be aware that there is a lot of false information available.